Mimicking Fasting

All the Benefits of Fasting
Without the Pain!

By

ODELIA ROSIE

Mimicking Fasting: All the Benefits of Fasting Without the Pain!

Publisher Contact

Skinny Bottle Publishing
books@skinnybottle.com

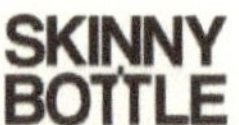

Introduction to Fasting

"The modern diet is the main reason why people all over the world are fatter and sicker than ever before"

— *Kris Gunnars, author and nutrition expert*

We don't need health professionals telling us that poor diets are hurting our health to be able to see the consequences of an unhealthy lifestyle.

If you walk down the street, most people you see have bulging bellies and generally look unhealthy. Perhaps you are also struggling with your weight and are looking for ways to shed some belly fat and become healthy again. Or, maybe you are not overweight but just feel unhealthy.

This book introduces a great new diet that will bring you heaps of health benefits and get you in great shape — The "Fasting Mimicking Diet."

The first part of this book will discuss how different diets can affect your health and the second part will explain and demonstrate the effects of the Fasting Mimicking Diet. You will discover the secrets of fasting and why it is good for your health. Lastly, I will introduce you to the Fasting Mimicking Diet, its benefits, what you should expect and how to go about it.

Diet and Your Health

It is common knowledge that a nutritious diet is vital to keeping one's health in top shape. Although most people are aware of this, only a small percentage will do something about it.

Sure, we know that a diet full of vegetables, fruits and lean protein is healthy, right? Still, most people would rather have ready-to-eat dinners, go to fast food restaurants and munch on "comfort foods," rather than prepare healthy and nutritious meals at home. Higher concentrations of sugar and larger portion sizes have caused people to increase their calorie intake. Unfortunately, when it comes to food, bigger and sweeter is not better.

But, what does this mean for you and why should you act right away?

Obesity on the Rise

The World Health Organization (WHO) defines overweight and obesity as "... an abnormal or excessive fat accumulation that may impair health." It is caused by "... an energy imbalance between calories consumed and calories expended." In simple terms, obesity is the result of individuals eating more calories than their body needs. Obesity is a not simply an aesthetic concern because it can lead to mental health issues and a reduced quality of life and obesity is the leading cause of deaths worldwide.

In their latest published statistics, the WHO reported that obesity worldwide has doubled since 1980. What was once a health concern only for high-income countries is an issue even for lower-income and middle-income nations. In fact, the WHO noted that there are a staggering 1.9 billion adults who are obese. Research conducted in 2011-2012 reported that In the U.S. alone, two-thirds of adults (68.6 percent) are either obese or overweight.

Obesity and its associated health implications have a significant economic impact on healthcare systems globally. Particularly, there is an increase in direct medical costs associated with preventing, diagnosing and treating all the issues related to obesity. Also, indirect costs can be substantial since most chronic diseases find their origins from obesity.

Effects of Obesity

It is not just about feeling good about your physical appearance and being able to wear your favorite jeans again. You should be conscious about your diet because an unhealthy diet can lead to many chronic illnesses. Obesity and poor nutrition put you at greater risk of developing a host of serious diseases. Some examples of these are:

High Blood Pressure — also known as hypertension. Obesity may cause difficulties for your heart, making it hard for it to pump blood throughout your body. According to health experts, eating too much salty, fried, sugary and junk foods can cause high blood pressure.

Heart Disease — high cholesterol foods, often common in Western diets, are a primary cause of heart disease. This illness is more prevalent in adults. The National Institute of Health (NHI) reports that over 610,000 people in the U.S. die from heart disease every year.

Type 2 Diabetes — according to the National Institute of Diabetes and Digestive Kidney Diseases, almost 80 percent of individuals who are overweight or obese have type 2 diabetes. This is not surprising since this illness is caused by a poor diet, sedentary lifestyle and having large amounts of visceral fat (also known as belly fat.) Type 2 diabetes is also associated with causing other illnesses such as heart disease, stroke and kidney disease.

Stroke — obesity can cause blood clots in arteries and blood vessels in the brain. Plaque build-up can cause a rupture of those blood vessels, leading to a stroke. Having high blood pressure also increases the risk of developing stroke.

Cancer — obesity increases the risk of developing several types of cancers such as breast, colon, kidney and gallbladder cancer.

If you are not convinced that obesity can degrade your health and even kill you, then you are good at lying to yourself.

Maybe you feel that you are off the hook because you are not overweight or obese. However, if you don't have a healthy diet, you may still be at risk of these chronic diseases — regardless of your weight.

If you act today, you can reduce the risk of these diseases and even lose a few pounds on the way. Fasting is one great method to achieve this goal.

Myths and misconceptions about obesity:

"I am overweight because I have a slow metabolism."

The truth is ... the speed of your metabolism does not vary to extremes. Just like the fact that you cannot lose weight without watching your diet and/or doing some physical activity; the same applies to weight gain. There is no way your body is adding fat mass if it is not provided with additional calories to use.

Adding some muscle mass to your frame will, in fact, increase your metabolism but not a drastic amount. Basically, the fitter you are, the more calories you burn during resting periods and even during exercise.

"I'm not overweight, I'm just big-boned."

Although it may be true that some individuals have bigger skeletal frames than others, that cannot be used as an excuse or explanation for high amounts of body fat. Having a large frame will only add 5-8 pounds on an adult and that weight will not increase with time.

"Childhood obesity is the parents' fault and caused only by eating junk food."

There's no need to point fingers or find something to blame when your kid is obese. As a family, your priority should be fixing the weight problem by working with your kids' caregivers. Junk food does not find its way into your home unless someone is buying it. The same can be said regarding visiting fast food restaurants; it should be a family responsibility to provide children with healthy eating options. Aside from food, we need to provide children with more opportunities for physical activity. Actually, taking walks with your children can be a great way for both of you to get some exercise. Remember to limit the number of hours your kids spend in front of the TV or playing video games as both of these will actually limit physical activity and encourage snacking.

What's the Fuss About Fasting?

You might have heard about fasting from your friends who have tried it or maybe you have read about the promised health benefits of fasting diets. But what makes a fasting diet different?

Fasting has been practiced by many cultures all over the world for centuries, often as a religious practice. Christians, Buddhists, Muslims and even Jews observe annual fasting days where believers abstain from food for a certain period of time as their way of penance and to connect with God.

However, through the years, fasting has evolved from only a religious practice to being used for health and medicinal purposes as well. Today, fasting is widely accepted as a health-improvement practice.

In recent years, there have been many types of fasting diets such as the 5:2 Diet, 16/8 Method and Eat-Stop-Eat. These diets involve skipping meals or dramatically reducing calorie intake for a number of days.

While there are experts who are hesitant to approve of these "extreme" diets, new research about fasting suggests that fasting is a safe and sound method for improving health improvement and dieting.

Benefits of Fasting

Improves your immunity — Scientists from the University of Southern California found that fasting for as little as three days can help regenerate the body's immune system. Fasting also helps the body to produce white blood cells, which helps in warding off infection.

Increases your metabolism — When one is in a state of fasting, there are several changes that happen in the body. Some of the changes are a significant drop in insulin levels, an increase in the levels of growth hormones and an increase in noradrenalin. These changes contribute to speeding up one's metabolism.

Helps you shed extra pounds — An increased metabolism causes the body to burn calories faster, which helps lose weight. Dramatically decreasing calorie consumption for a certain period of time also helps in shedding weight.

Fasting can be described as a way to "reset" the body and allow it to use fat as the body's primary source of fuel instead of sugar.

A 2014 study showed that individuals who underwent fasting reported having lost 4-7 percent of their visceral fat in the abdomen. This type of fat increases the risk of developing chronic illnesses.

Prevents type 2 diabetes — Studies have also shown that fasting helps to reduce insulin resistance, which also reduces blood sugar levels and lowers the risk of type 2 diabetes.

A study from the National Institute of Pharmaceutical Education and Research on diabetic rats showed that fasting helped in protecting against kidney damage, which is one of the primary consequences of diabetes.

Improves your heart health — Fasting lowers blood sugar levels and keeps blood pressure at healthy levels by reducing bad cholesterol. These effects help in decreasing the risk of heart disease. Heart disease is considered as one of the world's leading causes of death.

Helps prevent cancer — Research published in the *American Journal of Physiology* showed that fasting can help decrease the risk of developing cancer as it helps "starve" cancer cells. However, this research was conducted on mice, and studies about this particular outcome in humans have not yet been carried out.

Slows down aging — Research published in the *Journal of Nutritional*

Biochemistry and other research authored by the Louisiana State University Medical Center, showed that fasting helps improve the body's resistance to oxidative stress, which is a contributor to aging.

Supports brain health — The combined effects of fasting, such as the body's resistance to oxidative stress, reduced blood sugar levels, insulin resistance and reduced inflammation, all contribute to support the brain's health.

A study from the National Institute of Aging on rats reported that fasting can slow down the effects of Alzheimer's disease and reduce its severity.

Increases longevity — As one of the effects of fasting is to slow down aging; thus increasing your longevity. Two scientific studies suggest that in laboratory tests, fasting extended the lifespan of rats.

Fasting and Evolution

In early human history several thousand years ago, our ancestors survived on earing one meal a day after hunting or foraging for food. Nowadays, the stress of finding food and water has been reduced, with meats and produce readily available year-round at supermarkets worldwide. The question remains — has the human body evolved to the point where it really needs three meals a day?

In 2008, the National Institute on Aging published a study that addressed the effects of eating one meal a day on blood sugar and insulin sensitivity. Empirical evidence shows that evolution needs millions of years to change a simple gene. The question: From a biological point of view — are we as humans — ready to be consuming this abundance of food more than once a day?

The study did not focus on consuming fewer calories but on meal frequency. Results showed that by eating one heavy meal a day, participants exhibited a significant decrease in their fat mass and substantial increases in levels of LDL and HDL cholesterol. The participants were forced to eat a lot of food to match the calorie requirements of the participants eating three meals a day. (If this wasn't the case, most of them would have naturally eaten far fewer calories.)

The takeaway lesson is that the human body has not evolved to consume three meals a day and keep its digestive system running.

Therefore, the meal frequency our ancestors had is the most "natural" way for our body to function.

One example in history would be the average medieval Northern European peasants. They would generally have some sort of ale, bread or both for breakfast, then take a snack out into the fields with them and have their biggest meal around the afternoon when they were back home. This could have been eaten anytime between 2-6 p.m.

According to historians, there would not be another evening meal after this. In certain homes, peasants would just grab something light and quick as dinner. Back then, dinner was not thought of as the distinct meal as it is today. People also tended to consume their meals during daylight hours. This was not for any health-related reasons but because cooking, eating and washing were difficult to do in the dark.

Unless you were wealthy, you would not have a meal after dark. When electricity became available, upper-class households were the first to be able to eat as late as they wanted.

Methods of Fasting

Over the years, different fasting methods have sprung up to help individuals achieve their health goals. Some of the most popular fasting diets were:

5:2 Diet — In this diet, one would stick to their normal diet for five days and then restrict the food consumed to 25 percent of their normal calorie intake for the two remaining days of the week. During the fasting days, the average consumption would be 500 calories for women and 600 for men. However, it was recommended to use a calorie counter to estimate the calories that a particular body type needed.

You could stay on the diet for as long as you want and even make it your lifestyle. Some dieters switched to having only one day of fasting (6:1) after they reached their weight goal.

Alternate-Day Fasting (AFD) — This was an extreme style of fasting, suitable for people who could stick to a strict meal regimen. As the name implies, the diet required that one fasts every other day and go back to a normal diet between the fasting days (24 hours of non-fasting; 24 hours of fasting.) Like the 5:2 diet, during the "fasting days," the aim was to consume only 25 percent of the normal caloric intake in 24 hours which could be divided into three small meals.

Eat-Stop-Eat — This is another type of fasting that posed a challenge to many. Unlike the AFD which restricts consumption to 25 percent, the Eat-Stop=Eat method required that the dieter not consume any food within 24 hours.

16/8 Method — While the 5:2 Diet divided fasting and non-fasting days in a week, the 16/8 method divided the day into 16 hours of fasting and 8 hours of eating. This was one of the easiest diets to stick to because you only had to skip meals like breakfast or dinner. For example, if you ate breakfast at 8 a.m., you had until 4 p.m. to eat other meals. After a p.m., you had to fast until 8 a.m. the following day.

Fasting and Our Body

Upon waking up in the morning, your body has been fasting for 6-8 hours (more or less depending on when your last meal was and how long you have slept.) Because of this, your insulin level is low and your body is just starting to move into a state of fasting.

The worst thing for your metabolic system at this stage is food! This would cause your insulin levels to spike and immediately put a halt to any fat burning that has begun. A wiser choice would be to postpone any meal for a few hours in order to give your body time to enter the state of fasting. To be more precise, it's usually consuming carbohydrates that would create this insulin spike and shut off your fat-burning process.

Aside from not losing body fat, insulin is a lipogenic hormone, meaning that its secretion will drive the body into a "fat storage mode" instead. A spike of insulin is usually followed by hunger after a few hours, which continues the cycle of eating multiple meals per day. This may sound difficult, as most of us grew up dependent on carbohydrates, especially in the morning but this has never been the most appropriate fuel for our bodies.

The same evolution studies that have shown that humans have always been hunter-gatherers, tell us that instead of consuming a large breakfast in the morning, they would go hunt and gather to eat a big meal later in the day. Modern society has provided us with the worst options in terms of staying healthy. We are conditioned to eat frequently (up to six small meals a day) to maximize our fat-burning and to avoid going into starvation mode at all costs.

The truth is, starvation needs at least 3-4 days to start taking its toll on the body and there has not yet been anyone preaching a 4-day fasting diet. In order to burn fat optimally, you want to spend enough time fasting and then consume a big meal to prevent any starvation.

Scientists agree that a healthy person without any underlying medical conditions can fast for long periods of time without the risk of hypoglycemia. Almost all episodes of hypoglycemia or low blood sugar in healthy individuals are driven from consuming too many carbohydrates.

Fasting Mimicking Diet to the Rescue

Although the methods we discussed in the previous chapter are shown to be effective in providing the benefits of fasting, some people find compliance difficult. These methods require staying on the diet for extended periods in order to see and feel the benefits. If done wrong, these fasting diets could lead to adverse effects such as malnourishment and bodily dysfunctions. This is where the Fasting Mimicking Diet (FMD) comes to the rescue.

Anecdote

The benefits of the fasting-mimicking diet are far-reaching in medical field. For most of us, it is a great way to achieve the healthy weight and ideal figure that you have always dreamed of.

If you have considered FMD as a dietary therapy for controlling obesity, you certainly aren't alone. A lot of people are now beginning to rely on this approach as it makes it easy to diet without actually starving yourself. Among all the FMD experiences lies the story of Ian.

Ian was an extremely obese person and had left practically no stones unturned to lose weight. Sadly, nothing had worked on him so far. He weighed no less than 245 pounds when he first turned towards FMD. With a 50-in. waist and 38 percent body fat, he was at a very high risk of diabetes.

Starting FMD was definitely not easy for Ian. He was obese and disappointed in the very idea that food modifications were ever going to help him lose weight. However, he started FMD with the very last bits of hope that he still clung to. Ian went through three cycles of strict FMD and to his surprise, his body responded quite well. Not only did he shed pounds but also considerably improved his blood glucose, blood pressure and C-reactive proteins (an indicator of inflammation in the body.)

The improvements were not huge, possibly because he would turn to a high-sugar, high-fat and high-starch diet in between his cycles — which would ultimately lead to weight gain.

Considering the high risk of disease that Ian was constantly exposed to, it was suggested that he go through four cycles of the

FMD diet, all back-to- back, but under strict medical supervision. Most fasting clinics successfully make their patients go through a 200-calorie diet per day for up to four weeks without resulting in any serious consequences. So, it was perfectly safe for Ian to follow the FMD diet for three weeks by consuming 750 calories on a daily basis under a doctor's supervision.

FMD worked wonders for Ian who lost more than 30 pounds and a considerable amount of abdominal fat. His list of achievements also included a major boost in energy and overall well-being. Even after a year of going through FMD cycles, he has successfully maintained his weight. In his own words, Ian said, "FMD has literally turned my world upside down. It has miraculously helped me get healthy again when I had lost all hopes of recovery."

Ian was particularly impressed by the additional effect that came with FMD, the mental clarity that he started experiencing shortly after he started following the diet plan.

It is worth mentioning here that FMD plans involving two or more cycles must only be considered when period cycling has failed to produce any remarkable effects. Multiple FMD cycles need to be performed after the approval of a medical doctor. Moreover, a doctor, preferably the one holding a specialist degree in prolonged fasting therapies, must also carefully monitor you throughout your journey. This approach comes with potential side effects if the directions are not followed carefully. Some of these side effects include a drastic drop in blood glucose or blood pressure, in addition to malnourishment arising due to deficiency of vital minerals, nutrients and vitamins.

FMD may also generate a number of drug interactions, making the prolonged fasting approaches dangerous for certain groups, such as those on insulin therapy. Another related concern is combining the major weight loss and major weight gain — especially during cycling. A number of scientific studies have indicated that major weight loss during a FMD cycle, followed by a major weight gain in-between the cycles, can increase the risk of disease in both normal individuals as well as heart patients. It is also important to note that FMD is a tool that doctors use for the management of obesity and requires medical supervision.

The Fasting Mimicking Diet

FMD, a relatively new addition to the category of periodic diets, was introduced in mid-2015 by bio-gerontologist and cell biologist Dr. Valter Longo of the University of California (National Institute for Aging.) This study showed that FMD can mimic and yield the same effects and benefits of fasting.

The study was published by *Cell Metabolism.* It was a three-tier study that showed FMD's effects after tests on yeast, mice and humans.

Through testing on yeast, researchers could observe the effects of FMD on a cellular level. The mice tests, on the other hand, were done by having two cycles of FMD (lasting for four days) every month, followed by the mice's normal diet between the FMD days. The control group had the same consumption of calories as the FMD group to show that the effects of FMD were not due to restricting calories alone. Testing on the mice started when they were middle-aged (which was at 16 months.)

Human testing was conducted on 38 healthy adults, of which 19 were assigned to the FMD group. Those in the FMD group were given a plant-based diet (34-54 percent of their normal calorie intake) that was designed to mimic or achieve the effects of fasting. The diet still provided the vitamins and minerals the body needed as nourishment (9-10 percent protein, 34-47 percent carbohydrates and 44-56 percent fat) minimizing the "burden" of fasting.

The study provided the following specific types of foods:

1. Scientifically designed instant vegetable-based soup

2. Energy bars

3. Energy drinks

4. Kale chips

5. Chamomile tea

6. Vegetable supplement formula tablets

Participants were instructed to follow the FMD for five straight days every month for three months (which is equal to three cycles) and then go back to their usual diets after five days of FMD.

Effects of FMD

The effects of the FMD during and after testing were significant. Periodic fasting tests on yeast showed an increase in lifespan and increase in stress resistance which could also contribute to longevity.

The mice showed more promising results. The mice which started the FMD during their middle age had an extended lifespan. Mice in the control group had an average lifespan of 25.5 months, while those in the FMD group lived an average of 28.3 months. Researchers also noted that FMD could boost the mice's immune system, reduce inflammation, reduce visceral fat, prevent bone mineral density loss, reduce the incidence of cancer and most interestingly, improve the cognitive capacity in older mice.

Finally, the effects of FMD on humans became obvious right after the first cycle of the diet. It was reported that after the first month, the glucose levels of the FMD participants were reduced to 11 percent. The levels remained low even after going back to their normal diet, which came as a surprise to the researchers. Humans who underwent the FMD had increased ketone levels and reduced levels of the IGF-1 hormone (which is related to aging and cancer susceptibility.)

To summarize, the study clearly shows that FMD can indeed provide the same benefits of a usual fasting method. Specifically, the FMD can:

Speed up metabolism

FMD delivers enough nutrients to your body to stimulate the metabolism into becoming an efficient fat-burning machine. Fasting incorrectly can do the opposite, particularly when vital nutrients are missing. FMD is a healthy way to boost your metabolism by making sure that the digestive system and nutrient delivery processes are working at optimal rates. This will not only help you in reducing body fat but will also help detoxify your circulation system of all of the bad waste accumulated through years of unhealthy eating.

Rejuvenate and improve the immune system

The concept of boosting your immunity is enticing but remains a mystery for many. Balance and harmony are what is needed to boost your immune system. The immune system is an ever-evolving system that has to keep adapting to new risks and dangers. The most important vitamins that can improve our immune system's response are vitamins C and E. Vitamin C is the biggest booster for the immune system but it works in conjunction with vitamin E, a powerful antioxidant. Both vitamins are usually considered partners. Vitamin E is the main defense system against oxidative stress in the body but it is usually quickly depleted from its active components. This is where vitamin C comes into play. The role of Vitamin C is to regenerate vitamin E, so by consuming an adequate amount of both, we are ensuring that the immune system works to the fullest capacity.

Improve cognitive capacity, which prevents cognitive decline

Fasting has lots of positive effects on the brain and this can be seen through all of the positive neurochemical changes that occur in our brain when we follow a diet similar to FMD. Improvement in the cognitive function and stress resistance, elevation of neurotrophic factors and a decrease in inflammation are some of the proven benefits from this diet.

This is because FMD can be thought of as a challenge to your brain. The response to stimuli is the formation of stress response pathways to make sure our brain can cope with the risk induced by this stress. It's the same concept as building muscles; we add stress to our muscles by lifting heavy weight and the response is an increase in the muscle size. In the brain, a response to FMD is an increase of neurotrophic factors (special proteins in the brain) and strengthening of neuron synapses.

Help lower cancer risk

Human trials have shown that patients receiving chemotherapy while on a fasting diet (unintentionally) had similar results to cell count studies performed on mice. Fasting cycles in mice turned on a regenerative switch, modified the signaling pathways and promoted many stem cells. These cells are directly responsible for generating many cells within the immune system. One possible explanation for this was that when fasting, the body will cut down on unnecessary energy expenditure by recycling many of the immune cells that may be damaged. Fasting, therefore, improves the white blood cell count which translates into better immunity. Now for chemotherapy patients, that meant a quicker recovery but for healthy individuals, this provided them with a lower cancer risk. Another observation was the reduction of the PKA enzyme, which has been long-linked to aging and certain types of cancer.

Decrease inflammation, which also prevents the illnesses that are caused by it

Inflammation, by definition, is the progressive destruction of tissues. Depending on the location of these tissues, inflammation can sometimes be fatal. Inflammation is thought to be the cause of many diseases and by controlling inflammation, we can prevent many illnesses and diseases from progressing or even occurring. In 2015, Yale University scientists showed the exact way fasting is able to tame inflammation. The study demonstrates the compound β-hydroxybutyrate (BHB) and its ability to directly inhibit a complex set of proteins known as NLRP3. The NLRP3 is responsible for the inflammation behind many chronic diseases. BHB is produced when the body is in a fasting state or after bouts of high-intensity workouts. When BHB was introduced in mice suffering from inflammation, signs of improvement were quickly visible.

Lower blood sugar levels, which may prevent type 2 diabetes

We have discussed the effects of lowering insulin spikes in the morning but the fact remains that reducing insulin spikes at any time of the day is helpful in keeping blood sugar levels down. Type 2 diabetes is a condition in the body which keeps blood sugar high. It is generally caused by the body being sensitive to changes in insulin. In healthy individuals, the release of insulin from the pancreas is enough to stabilize blood sugar levels. Constantly elevated blood sugar levels from bad dieting and obesity can lead to placing the pancreas under a huge amount of stress. As the years pass by, the risk of impairment in the amount of insulin produced by the pancreas increases, leading to diabetes. Type 2 diabetes is diagnosed when the insulin produced by the body is no longer able to maintain a normal baseline blood sugar level. Unfortunately, there is no cure for type 2 diabetes. So, by keeping our blood sugar level low, we are protecting our body from developing type 2 diabetes and the many health complications that arise as a result.

Reduce visceral fat, which is seen as a risk for developing heart disease, stroke, hypertension, and cancer

Since the 1980s, studies have shown that there is a correlation between visceral fat and many metabolic diseases. Individuals with high visceral fat are at a higher risk of cardiovascular disease. Visceral fat is different from subcutaneous fat. The fat that is just below the skin is known as subcutaneous fat but visceral fat is more dangerous. This is the fat mass found in the abdomen and around certain vital organs.

Improve longevity

Human cells react to fasting similarly as they do to exercise. In other words, when placed under stress, the cells try to create some changes to extend their lifespan. Aside from cellular level changes, the fact that FMD can prevent many diseases, is a way to increase longevity.

What makes FMD special is that these benefits can be obtained faster and with less effort. Traditional fasting is often associated with pains such as headaches and sleeping problems. FMD participants reported these side effects too, but they were few and mild at worst. They also reported no problems sleeping.

"It's not a typical diet because it isn't something you need to stay on," says Dr. Longo in a published interview online. According to him, FMD can be repeated every three-to-six months for most individuals, depending on your health and your waist measurement (visceral fat.)

For the majority of people, food and emotion are strongly linked. Changing our habits is not as easy as it sounds, especially when it creates psychological chaos. This is why it is hard to change old habits and to stick to a new regimen. The challenge here is to change your perspective about fasting by changing your mental state. Yes, the first day might be confusing a bit and you will feel uneasy but usually by the third day there will be a shift in energy and the body will function optimally again.

Who May Benefit From FMD?

One of the most common questions that people have regarding FMD is who should try it?

FMD can be safely followed by all the healthy adults between the ranges of 18-to-70 years and are of normal weight. This long-term fasting plan might be incompatible with a number of genetic mutations, however. If you are going through an FMD cycle and start experiencing side effects other than slight tiredness, weakness or a headache, it is important for you to contact the doctor. Drinking a small quantity of fresh fruit juice is also warranted for immediate relief.

Who may NOT Benefit from FMD?

FMD certainly has its own set of benefits; however, this dietary approach is certainly not recommended for everyone. Certain groups are strictly prohibited to follow FMD which include:

- Pregnant females
- Underweight people as they usually suffer from anorexia or have an extremely low body mass index (BMI)
- People above the age of 70, unless they are in extremely good health — even then, it's mandatory to begin FMD with a doctor's approval
- Any person who is fragile
- People who are suffering from any disease of the liver or kidney
- People who are victims of pathologies, unless they have been deemed fit for FMD by a specialized doctor. In people

suffering from serious illness such as diabetes, cancer, cardiovascular, neurodegenerative or an autoimmune disease, it is extremely important to consult with and get approval from a disease specialist in addition to a dietitian expert in FMD. The use of FMD approach for the treatment of certain diseases must be limited to the clinical trials unless there is no other alternative option left and the patient is not in a condition to wait for the FDA approval.

- Patients who are taking medicines must not start FMD without getting an approval from their doctor with an input from a dietitian who specializes in FMD. It might be possible to successfully combine FMD with a lot of medicines without producing any side effects. However, there have been instances of fatal outcomes without proper medical oversight.

- Patients suffering from hypertension and are taking anti-hypertensive medications. Such patients must never undertake this approach without discussing it with a specialist first.

- People suffering from certain rare genetic mutations that block their body's capacity to perform gluconeogenesis (*i.e.* production of glucose from amino acids and glycerol.)

- Athletes, especially during competition or training sessions. A routine involving high muscular effort needs high levels of glucose that are typically not found in the blood during a FMD cycle. This can ultimately increase the risk of fainting.

Warnings Related to FMD

In addition to following the regular instructions regarding FMD, it is also important to keep some warnings in mind regarding everyday life. These warnings are not just there to keep you cautious but will make your transformation journey considerably easier.

1. Always remember that FMD is never suitable to follow in association with any medication that targets your blood sugar levels, such as insulin. This combination can prove lethal for you. By the end of a normal FMD cycle, you still might be sensitive to insulin and may also have a lesser than normal amount of sugar in your blood. Using FMD for a patient suffering from diabetes can be particularly dangerous. Therefore, it is advised for such patients to only adopt this diet as a part of some clinical trial.
2. Even if you are a fan of hot showers that last for hours, never combine it with FMD, particularly if it is hot outside. This type of combination can increase your risk of fainting.
3. Always be careful while driving. It is better if you do not drive altogether unless you figure out how this approach is affecting you.
4. It is always better to undergo FMD while there is another person present around you for support, especially if something unfortunate happens.

How Often Must You Undertake FMD?

This decision relies on several factors and must be made in consultation with a registered doctor and a dietitian. However, some broad guidelines for a general overview on how often FMD can be followed are:

1. Once a month by people who are obese or overweight and have at least two identified risk factors for cancer, diabetes, neurodegenerative or cardiovascular disease
2. Once every two months by people with normal weight and at least two identified risk factors for cancer, diabetes, neurodegenerative or cardiovascular disease
3. Once every three months by people with normal weight and at least one identified risk factor for cancer, diabetes, neurodegenerative or cardiovascular disease
4. Once every four months by patients in good health who follow a good diet plan but are not physically active
5. Once every six months by the healthy patients having an ideal diet and are regularly engaging in physical activity

Following the Fasting Mimicking Diet

Learning about the results of FMD and how it can provide you the benefits of fasting will quickly entice you to go on the diet. But where do you start?

L-Nutra is a company established in 2009 by nutrition experts who came up with a product called ProLon (http://l-nutra.com). This product provides contains the same foods as the FMD study. A single cycle of ProLon comes with four energy drink mixes, six energy bars, pouches of kale chips, capsules of oil, supplement tables, tea bags and 10 packets of FMD soup. These will be consumed in the first five days of the diet.

When is FMD Ideally Started?

A lot of people decide to go to FMD on a Sunday night. This allows them to end it following Friday night. The decision is purely based on social interactions and hence, permits them to return to their transition diet by Friday night. This can then be followed by returning to a normal night on Saturday.

FMD must never be started abruptly. There must be a preparatory phase that should begin approximately one week before you properly switch to FMD. During this preparatory phase, you must ideally consume 0.36 grams of protein per pound of your body weight on a daily basis. The preferred sources of protein should be fish and vegetables. The preparatory phase also includes taking omega-3 multivitamin supplements twice during the week.

DAY ONE

The first day is a transition from your normal diet to FMD. On day one, you can have 1,090 calories in total — an easy start! You can have tea and an energy bar for breakfast. You should also take the oil capsule.

Don't forget to drink lots of water during the diet to avoid dehydration. You can munch on an energy bar for your lunch or your afternoon snack. And finally, you can have soup for dinner with the kale chips.

DAY TWO-DAY FIVE

From day two onwards you can only have 725 calories per day for the remaining fasting days. Your meals will include the energy drinks, vegetable soup, energy bars, kale chips and of course, the supplements that are provided.

Although you may feel that these foods are not enough, remember that they are designed to provide the energy and nutrients that our body needs. That's why those who have tried FMD have reported no drop in their energy levels even though they consumed fewer calories.

DAY SIX

Congratulations! You just finished the first FMD cycle. Give yourself a pat on the back for a job well done. Before you go ahead and get back to your normal diet, you should allow a 12-hour transition period (or longer) with a liquid or soft diet. Consider having soup, fruit juices or veggies. This will ensure a smooth transition to your normal diet.

DAY SEVEN

Now, you can go back to your normal diet. No, you do not have to count calories or skip meals. However, it is strongly recommended to stay within reasonable calorie-consumption bounds. Even though FMD is proven to work, it doesn't mean that you should start bingeing on high cholesterol, sugary and greasy foods after the first cycle is over. Always try to include veggies, fruits and lean protein in your diet.

Although FMD is proven to be effective, if you have existing health conditions, you should always advise your doctor before trying this diet.

What Goes on in Your Body During the First Days of FMD?

First, let us discuss how your metabolism operates during your normal dieting days, right up to your first day on FMD.

In modern times, carbohydrates have become our main source of energy. When consumed in high amounts (around 50 percent of total intake on average) they will cause a spike in blood sugar level. This level must be maintained at around 70-to-100 mg/100ml. Insulin is the hormone that keeps our blood sugar in check. After food is digested, our pancreas produces insulin to bring blood sugar down to satisfactory levels. This works by simply storing insulin in the liver and the muscle tissue. But when excessive amounts of carbohydrates are consumed, the only way to get rid of the extra blood sugar is by transforming it into fatty acids through multiple synthesis reactions.

When we start FMD, we disrupt the whole process of using carbohydrates as our main source of energy. In the first few hours — due to lack of consumed foods rich in carbohydrate — the body is going to dip into its storage reserves in the liver. Stored sugar will then be released to keep our blood sugar within the normal levels. After a few more hours, our body will detect storage depletion and start acting to maintain an energy flow to the vital organs. The next logical source of energy is now fat.

After being in the fasted state for more than 12 hours, two hormones known as epinephrine and norepinephrine are released. These are known as the stress hormones and their job is to get the body out of this stressful situation. Up until now, our body has been used to having carbohydrates as a source of energy. Once depleted, the panic switch is hit and the stress hormones are released. The job of these stress hormones is to enhance the release of fat from the adipose tissue in order to transform it into energy.

By day two of the FMD diet, the lack of carbohydrate intake has geared your endocrine system to tap into its stored energy for immediate use. Glucose stored in the liver is already depleted but that does not mean that we are only running on fat. The muscle tissue also has some glucose stored and the epinephrine and norepinephrine are reaching out for it. At the start of day two, the body is now running on a combination of mainly fat oxidation and the remaining glucose stores in the muscle mass. This is why for some individuals, day two is the biggest challenge as your body is literally draining its last glucose storage.

On day three, the magic is starting to happen. By now, your body has depleted all its glucose stores and is looking for efficient ways to melt down those fatty cells and transform them into usable energy. A process called "de novo synthesis" is responsible for transforming those fat deposits into glucose. Another source is the protein found in the muscle mass, which will start degrading in hope of being turned into fuel. Lucky for the body, FMD lasts only five days, so no real harm is done on the muscle tissue.

By the end of day three, the body has switched from using carbohydrates as its main source of energy to ketones. Ketones are molecules synthesized from fatty acids that are capable of converting into a fuel source after a series of complex reactions.

For the next two days, more and more ketones are produced, using mainly body fat stores and keeping the body in a state of ketosis (using ketones for energy.)

There you go! You have successfully completed the five days of the FMD and proved to your body that carbohydrates are not the only source of energy that can be used to sustain itself. Another process that usually starts around day five is the increase of growth hormones levels. These hormones are meant to limit the amount of muscle and protein lost. This, in turn, will increase the use of fatty acids and ketones as primary sources of energy.

Another main concern during any fasting is micronutrients. This is why the FMD is not void of nutrients; you are still consuming food with minimal calories but packed with nutrients. Potassium, sodium and phosphorus are three essential micronutrients that the body has to preserve and making good food choices during these five days is important for staying healthy.

Another thing to remember is on day six — don't start bingeing on food from the second you wake up. You need to transition yourself back to your normal food intake. Spend the first 12 hours slowly increasing your food intake to give your functions time to recover. Your pancreas and liver need to gradually shift into a different physiological process; this is to avoid getting bouts of hyperglycemia which can sometimes be accompanied with nasty symptoms, such as diarrhea or nausea.

Now repeating this cycle every month is a sure way to train your body into shifting towards a better blood sugar control, a stronger immune system and reduced risk of various chronic diseases.

What Should You Expect From the FMD?

FMD is without a doubt, a great way to achieve your desired body weight and fight different health-related problems. Yet, people need to be mentally prepared for what this approach is going to bring along with it. For this purpose, you need to familiarize yourself with both the positive and negative aspects of the FMD.

Negative Effects

It is common for some people to feel weakness at several points during the FMD. For others, the approach may seem energizing. Sometimes, patients may also complain of headaches of mild to moderate intensity during the FMD cycle. This side effect can be managed by day five and is usually eliminated by the end of second of the third cycle of FMD.

During the initial days of FMD, some people feel extreme hunger. However, there is nothing to worry about as this unpleasant feeling is greatly reduced by the fourth or fifth day. Additionally, this effect does not reappear as you move into your second and third FMD cycle.

Sometimes, a slight backache may make occur during the regular FMD cycle. This backache usually resolves as the person switches back to a normal diet.

Positive Effects

Some of the most famous positive effects that the users are guaranteed to experience during FMD are a significant reduction in abdominal fat, a boost in stem cell production and a decrease in the risk factors for several diseases. However, the positive effects of the FMD are not confined to these.

Yes, there is a lot more to FMD than you are told. FMD promises to give you glowing skin which many of you refer to as a "younger-looking skin." It enhances your mental focus and develops an ability for you to resist bingeing when you return to a normal diet.

A lot of people are successfully able to reduce their daily consumption of calories and sugars. Moreover, they are less prone to consume excessive amounts of alcohol, coffee and desserts. This is what changes their entire eating habits and transforms their lives permanently.

Now that you have a clear understanding about what FMD is and how it affects your body, it is time to go into detail about how this diet can help you in prevention, delay, treatment and even reversal of certain diseases. The link between FMD and various diseases is important to understand and explore, especially if you are at a high risk or suffering from diabetes, cancer, cardiovascular disorders, autoimmune problems and neurodegenerative diseases such as Alzheimer's disease.

FMD AND DIABETES

The best way to prevent diabetes and significantly lower its risk is to maintain an ideal weight. Studies conducted on human and animal models have shown that a strict calorie-restricted diet can prevent diabetes completely in monkeys or cause a dramatic decrease in the fasting blood glucose levels and abdominal fat in humans and make it impossible for these people to ever develop diabetes.

However, following a strict calorie-restricted diet is not possible. A huge number of people are not able to maintain a diet with a 30 percent calorie restriction. These people are not willing to give up on most of the foods they relish. Some of them do not want to lose large quantities of muscle mass, while others just do not want to be too thin. All of these concerns are valid as they are unavoidable in a person who is on calorie-restriction regimen for a long time. Additionally, a lot of studies have indicated that calorie restriction cannot decrease the levels of fasting blood glucose in obese people as it can in people with average weight. Therefore, it is necessary to formulate suitable strategies that are well-suited to most of the people.

In the following section, I present both the everyday dietary changes and the periodic fasting-mimicking diets that can be adopted to prevent and help reverse diabetes.

By far, two short-term approaches that involve some kind of fasting have been found to be effective in the management of diabetic risk factors. One of them has been formulated by Dr Michelle Harvie (University of Manchester) and further modified by a journalist named Michael Mosley. The approach is named as "5:2 Diet" and involves overweight subjects who consume 500 to 600 calories two times a week for up to six months. This approach has been able to markedly reduce their abdominal fat and improve insulin sensitivity.

The diet has been recorded to have a limited effect on the blood glucose of overweight patients which indicates that diabetic patients need longer treatment durations.

The biggest advantage of this diet is that it does not involve close monitoring and needs minimal medical supervision. The disadvantage, on the other hand, is that most of the obese patients suffering from diabetes may find it tough to follow this diet on a long-term basis, mainly because it requires strict dietary restriction twice weekly.

A concern that still needs to be addressed regarding this diet is that switching between a 500-calorie and a 2000-calorie diet might stimulate metabolic disturbances and sleep disorders that resemble jet lag. Nevertheless, thousands of people have tried the 5:2 diet, — especially to lose weight —and many of them have reported positive effects.

The doctors must be the ones to decide whether or not their patients need this diet incorporated into their regular treatment plans.

The other diet plan that has been used successfully to handle diabetes is the FMD approach.

FMD as the Treatment for Diabetes

Diabetes drugs may either activate or interfere with the normal working of enzymes that lower blood glucose. However, these drugs do not directly target the main reason causing diabetes. FMD can be helpful in this regard. The results of various clinical trials being conducted have produced promising results. These trials concluded that undergoing 5-day FM cycles three times month can allow your body to mimic fasting (consumption of 750 to 1100 calories on a daily basis.) This has successfully reduced some of the major risk factors for metabolic syndromes like diabetes.

Metabolic Reprogramming as a Treatment for Diabetes

Scientists usually tend to be cautious in using the word "cure" since it seems like an exaggeration. However, in some cases, the patients with diabetes type 2 can actually be cured by combining the medical interventions with suitable dietary modifications. This is also true for a large share of pre-diabetics. This obviously does not mean that every diabetic person can be cured or that it is easy for these patients to follow this approach.

However, the data from animal and human studies have strongly suggested that a lot of people who undergo chronic dietary modifications such as FMD can eventually be cured of type 2 diabetes. This is particularly true if the treatment begins right after the initial diagnosis when the pancreas is still functional.

It is important to take note that combining diabetes drugs and FMD is extremely dangerous and must only be done as a part of clinical trials. It must also be noted that even though all the clinical data successfully indicate the high potential of FMD and similar approaches for the treatment of diabetes, this still needs to be proven in a large randomized clinical trial and must be approved by the FDA. Only then, can it be prescribed to patients as an alternative to the standard care for diabetes. However, these dietary interventions can still be adopted as a support to the FDA-approved therapies.

If you are at an extremely high risk of diabetes or are suffering from it, it is encouraged that you talk to your doctor and change your everyday diet right now. This dietary modification will serve as a preventive measure as well as a treatment intervention.

Various studies have indicated that FMD can reverse diabetes, but how does it do this?

There are a number of proposed reasons:

Reduction of the Liver and Abdominal Fat

FMD can push the body into a high fat-burning state, primarily with the help of visceral or abdominal fat. Liver fat, which plays a central role in the promotion of diabetes and other related conditions, is also utilized in this process. In clinical trials, it has been observed that the mice that undergo two cycles of FMD per month while matching the monthly intake of the mice that were eating normally tended to lose weight. This highly suggests the body's fat-burning state continue, even when the person has returned to a normal diet.

Promotion of Fat Loss Without Losing Muscle

In the human trials carried out to test FMD, it was observed that the obese participants lost around 9 pounds after going through three FMD cycles. In the overweight patients, the average amount of weight lost was around 4.5 pounds. At the same time, the negligible loss observed in lean body mass suggested that FMD can help reduce fat without any significant loss of muscle.

Autophagy and Cell Regeneration/ Renewal

FMD has a tendency to flush out bad cells by triggering old and damaged cells to reset or diet. At the same time, it can spur regeneration inside the cell — a process known as *autophagy* —in which the cell destroys itself. All these processes ultimately lead to rejuvenation and regeneration.

In mice, this process has been demonstrated to occur in different systems such as the muscle, brain, blood, pancreas and liver. In humans, the data extracted from various clinical trials suggest that the same regenerative process occurs. Healthy subjects with low levels of blood glucose or blood pressure experienced minimal or no change after going through FMD cycling in order to protect their glucose levels from dipping dangerously low.

At the same time, the effects of FMD on prediabetics and diabetics were considerably strong. The diet was seen to affect their blood glucose, blood pressure and several other risk factors. These results from human trials, together with the information collected from animal experiments, suggest that FMD triggers regeneration, rejuvenation or both process in the body. If the muscle cells responding poorly to insulin are regenerated, rejuvenated or repaired, their normal function can definitely be stored.

FMD and Pancreatic Regeneration

In a recently published scientific trial, the researchers have shown that the cycles of FMD can not only improve insulin function but can also stimulate the regeneration of pancreatic beta-cells responsible for the production of insulin. It treated both type 1 and type 2 diabetes along with all of its symptoms in mice with not enough pancreatic capability to generate insulin.

Surprisingly, the FMD led to the activation of a number of pancreatic genes that are normally activated during the fetal development period. This suggested that the FMD approach can initiate a natural and coordinated regenerative response resulting in new, highly functional beta cells which produce insulin and normalize body glucose.

Death in people undergoing a chronic fasting diet is quite rare and has only occurred when the diet has been associated with insulin use. Some of the patients died from combining their fasting diet with insulin injections, mainly because insulin works poorly in patients with diabetes and fasting can reverse this effect. The same insulin injection that tends to decrease glucose levels to a healthy level in a diabetic person, can result in a much more impulsive loss in a diabetic person who is fasting at the same time. This ultimately leads to hypoglycemic shock and in some cases, death can occur.

FMD and Cardiovascular Diseases

As per the American Heart Association, cardiovascular disease is a broad category which includes stroke, coronary heart disease, high blood pressure, coronary failure and different arterial diseases. Cardiovascular disease is said to kill over 801,000 people in the U.S.

each year. This means that 1 out of every 3 deaths occurring in the U.S. is due to a cardiovascular disease. In addition,, more than 92 million people in the U.S. are living with some type of cardiovascular disease.

The costs related to the treatment and the loss of productivity are said to be around $316 billion. The statistical analysis clearly indicates that medicines and other interventions being prescribed for cardiovascular disease are not very effective.

Luckily, FMD has shown a new ray of hope in this regard. This particular approach is said to have the potential for reducing the incidence as well as the progression of cardiovascular diseases. Two lengthy studies involving monkeys are the greatest proof that supports this treatment. Various human studies have also indicated the power of FMD and other dietary interventions in combating this global problem.

The FMD approach is particularly helpful in combatting cardiovascular diseases. This is because it does not focus on blocking the activity of enzymes that play a significant role in the progression of these diseases. In fact, the goal of this treatment is to stimulate the ability of your body to promote cellular rejuvenation, protection and regeneration. These effects combine to improve the function and restore you to a healthy state.

As with diabetes, the effects of undergoing periodic FMD on the risk factors associated with cardiovascular disorders are exceptional; although larger clinical trials are still needed to confirm this. When the FMD approach was tested in humans, the subjects indicated a lower incidence of cardiovascular disease and a reduction in inflammation markers after only three cycles of diet. Moreover, no adverse side effects were seen during this period.

Other findings in these subjects included a reduction in the body weight as well as body mass but no reduction in lean mass was observed. Three cycles of FMD were carried out once a month. The cycles continued for five days, followed by a return to the normal diet. This routine caused a reduction in the abdominal circumference of up to 1.6 in. in all the participants.

In general, the FMD cycles were found to be more effective in individuals exposed to higher levels of risk factors as compared to the healthy individuals. For instance, the systolic blood pressure was reduced by 7 mmHg in participants with moderately elevated blood pressure. The triglycerides level in patients with hypertriglyceridemia were decreased by 25 mg/dL and the level of bad cholesterol or LDL was reduced by 22 mg/dL in patients at risk of cardiovascular diseases. Interestingly, three cycles of FMD successfully returned the levels of CRP (an inflammatory risk factor for cardiovascular disorders), to normal levels in the majority of subjects.

In another clinical study involving 100 participants, The FMD cycles significantly reduced the major markers or risk factors related to cardiovascular diseases, particularly in people who were at high risk. The results of FMD in relation to cardiovascular diseases include:

- Reduction in abdominal circumference and fat
- Major drop in CRP, an important inflammatory marker
- Reduction in the total cholesterol
- Decreased LDL cholesterol levels
- Lowered levels of triglycerides
- Reduction in the fasting blood glucose
- Decrease in both systolic and diastolic blood pressure

Neurodegenerative Diseases and the Role of FMD

The brain function and the damage inflicted upon it has been a scholarly focus of many researchers. The brain is commonly hit by diseases such as Parkinson's and Alzheimer's, that are devastating, not only to the sufferers but also to the people around them. This chapter will mainly focus on different diseases of the brain such as dementia and Alzheimer's disease and discuss how nutrition and FMD might affect their prevalence and progression. The studies targeting Parkinson's disease are limited and need further clinical research, however, it is highly hoped that FMD along with other dietary modifications, will be able to positively affect it.

Alzheimer's Disease

Alzheimer's disease majorly accounts for 60-80 percent of all types of dementias. The disease is characterized by a loss of memory that commonly interferes with the daily tasks. During the early stages of the disease, patients find it difficult to remember any newly-acquired information. Later on, disorientation occurs, followed by changes in mood and behavior. The patient becomes suspicious of his own family members and caretakers as he fails to recognize and remember them. As the memory loss progresses, the patient may even have a difficulty in walking, speaking and swallowing.

In the past, a great promise in fighting Alzheimer's disease was a vaccine that targeted a protein known as beta-amyloid. This protein tends to accumulate in the brain of a patient and cause main symptoms of this disease. Despite the high expectations and hopes, this strategy has been unable to produce effective results and a lot of laboratories are still in search of the perfect cure for this disease. The role of beta-amyloid in the development and progression of Alzheimer's disease is also suspicious now.

Even a delay of five years in the average age of the patient with an Alzheimer's diagnosis is capable of reducing the number of patients by almost half. This is because the onset of this disease occurs at an age where a lot of patients are prone to dying of another cause. Hence, Alzheimer's disease is a good candidate for the utilization of dietary interventions like FMD that has shown great effects on the process of aging and can delay the onset or progression of this disease.

FMD and Neurodegenerative Diseases

The major risk factor for neurodegenerative diseases such as Alzheimer's is aging. The incidence of this disease increases by over a hundredfold in a person age 60-95. Studies of mice have already provided a platform to understand Alzheimer's disease. The human genes leading to the development of this neurodegenerative disease are introduced into the genome of the mouse. The resulting the memory loss and learning deficits that occur in the patients are observed. It feels sad that the scientists need to sacrifice mice for identifying interventions for Alzheimer's disease but these preliminary tests are absolutely essential before the human testing officially begins.

Because of the animal testing, the official clinical trials for the use of FMD in prevention as well as treatment of Alzheimer's disease, have officially begun. The preliminary studies involving investigations on how FMD acts on the cognitive performance in healthy participants revealed positive results. These promising results have formed the basis for possible correlation of Alzheimer's disease intervention to FMD.

The first attempt at delaying the onset of Alzheimer's disease involved regulation of the genes that accelerate the process of aging. For this purpose, "triple transgenic" mice were used having three mutated human genes that are strongly associated with the Alzheimer's disease. These genes include APP, tau and PS1 gene. Because Alzheimer's disease usually occurs after age 70, the scientists chose against the use of a chronic low-calorie diet even if it is proved to be effective. The elderly people would not be able to adopt it.

The scientists regulated the activity of two primary sets of genes that accelerate aging via tricking of cells. The mice used in the study were provided with a normal diet that was lacking in nine essential amino acids. These amino acids included threonine; methionine; leucine; isoleucine; lysine; phenylalanine; valine, tryptophan and arginine, and could not be produced naturally by the body. The mice were also provided with extra amounts of non-essential amino acids that can be produced by the human body; hence, they do not need to be obtained from the diet. In simpler terms, the test was similar to a regular diet with non-essential amino acids and a lesser amount of essential amino acids.

The mice began taking this diet at a young to middle age. The special diet was repeated every other week while alternating with a regular diet. The strong effect of this little change because obvious by a 75 percent reduction in the amount of cancer growth factor (IGF-1) and pro-aging factors in mice while they were still on diet.

The effects of this particular dietary intervention continued on the IGF-1 levels even after the mice resumed their normal diet. Even after a few months, the mice that had been placed on a protein-restricted diet showed better performance in several cognitive tests. This indicated that these mice were protected from the symptoms of the Alzheimer's disease.

These results particularly depict the true potential of nutritechnology. Understanding the true effects of food composition on certain pathways and genes can help develop therapeutic diets which are minimally disruptive yet strong enough to compete for the standard drug therapy. This concept is a little different than that of "nutraceuticals," which refers to food specially engineered to concentrate the levels of certain molecules with medical or biological significance. (For instance, the concentrated form of vitamin C derived from acerola is a nutraceutical.)

In another study, the mice had to undergo FMD in the form of four-day cycle twice every month. The mice started at middle age and it was noticed that as they approached old age, they had better memory as compared to mice belonging to control group. The performance improvement was observed in almost all of the tests such as motor coordination in both short- and long-term memory.

The FMD cycles are said to have strong effects on the genes that play a primary role in the process of aging, particularly of the brain. Researchers belonging to the U.S. National Institute on Aging have conducted numerous trials in this area and focused on alternate-day fasting. Receiving no food one day and resuming a normal diet the very next day caused the mice to show improvements in both memory and learning functions. The benefits were significantly visible in normal mice as well as those with Alzheimer's disease.

Dietary Modifications to Prevent Alzheimer's Disease

Periodic FMD is said to promote a longer and a healthier lifespan. Therefore, it is recommended for most people. However, this diet tends to provide very few calories and may not be suitable for people who are over the age of 70. So, what would be the basis of adopting a diet that prevents the initiation of Alzheimer's disease if the same dietary plan will cause a deficiency in the immune system or make the patient weak?

Therefore, before recommending a dietary intervention, it is important to weigh its potential to prevent or cure a disease against its potential to introduce side effects. The minimal risks of opting an FMD in a patient of 65 years can be justified if the person is at high risk of developing Alzheimer's disease. This approach must generally be considered up to the age of 70, or possibly for older ages, depending upon the capability of a person to prevent the muscle mass loss and the consensus of a neurologist.

Different studies have indicated that a calorie-districted diet can improve or even prevent the loss of muscle mass in animals of older age. This warrants further studies to check if periodic FMD can exert positive or negative effects on muscle mass as well as strength in the elderly.

Because of the availability of cheap and specific DNA tests, it is now easy to consider diets that are designed especially to prevent a certain disease in individuals. For instance, the APOE protein that carries cholesterol and the cholesterol-like molecules are available in three different forms. These forms include APOE2, APOE3 and APOE4. For certain people who have two copies of APOE4 genes, the risk of acquiring Alzheimer's disease rises up to 15 times. In the general population, the chances of developing Alzheimer's disease after the age of 85 is greater than 40 percent. In case an individual has two copies of APOE4 genes, the risk for this disease can increase to as high as 91 percent. Half of such individuals tend to acquire this disease as soon as they reach the age of 68.

People whose parents or grandparents are patients with Alzheimer's disease must continue genetic testing in order to determine if they possess these risk factors. If the tests are positive, they may wish to consult their doctor about pursuing certain dietary recommendations.

Aging and Autoimmune System

As humans age, the possibility of damage to and the consequent malfunctioning of the immune system increases. The white blood cells such as macrophages, T cells and neutrophils constitute a central part of immunity and produce various inflammatory factors. A lot of immune functions are modulated by these white blood cells — such as killing bacteria and viruses and damaged cells such as cancerous ones.

As you age in association with disease, the generation of the immune cells, as well as the inflammatory factors, gets disturbed. When this happens, the body suffers from inflammation even if it is not required. This results in a low level of systemic inflammation that involves the entire body. Sometimes, this inflammation leads to the development of a potent immunity against the normal cells and the molecules within. This results in *self-recognition*, a condition in which the immune system starts attacking different parts of its own body. This is exactly what happens in autoimmune diseases like type 1 diabetes, Crohn's disease, and multiple sclerosis.

One way to check whether you are suffering from systemic inflammation (a risk factor for several cardiovascular diseases and cancer), is to measure the amount of C-reactive protein (CRP) present in the blood. The liver normally produces CRP as a response to systemic inflammation. Studies have indicated that over one-third of U.S. adults suffer from systemic inflammation as measured by their CRP levels. However, a large majority of European and well as other populations are affected by it. Systemic inflammation in such individuals is usually an outcome of unhealthy behaviors, exposure to infection and obesity.

Since the Mediterranean diet is linked with a decreased risk of disease, a lot of Europeans believe that their diet essentially protects them. Unfortunately, even the strictest forms of the Mediterranean diet have only a limited number of useful effects on aging and progression of the disease. Moreover, the diet is not completely adopted —even in the Mediterranean areas — particularly because people are unaware of what it truly entails and because it is one of the strictest diet plans.

A recent analysis conducted worldwide has shown that 8-to-9 percent of the population has been diagnosed with one out of 29 major autoimmune diseases — type 1 diabetes, Crohn's disease, multiple sclerosis, lupus, psoriasis, polymyalgia and rheumatoid arthritis being the most common.

The number of newly diagnosed patients with autoimmune diseases has been on the rise for almost three decades. During the last decade, an alarming increase of 19 percent has been noticed in the prevalence of these diseases. The incidence of autoimmune diseases is said to be doubling every five years. A portion of this increase can be related to improved diagnosis and awareness; however, dietary and environmental factors are also thought to play a role.

Diet and Autoimmune Diseases

Obesity has been associated with many autoimmune diseases such as rheumatoid arthritis and multiple sclerosis. It has also been related to Crohn's disease and other autoimmune disorders of the gut. Because fat cells can produce inflammatory molecules such as IL-6 and TNF alpha, the link between obesity and the autoimmune diseases can be associated with abdominal fat. The fat that is accumulated in the abdomen, as well as other parts of the body, is capable of generating molecules that initiate immune responses and prompt the immune cells to work against other cells of the body.

Consumption of high levels of salt is also a primary contributor to autoimmune diseases. Salt promotes T cell activation, a primary culprit in a variety of autoimmune diseases. More studies are required to confirm the role played by sodium in autoimmune diseases but because it is also involved in the progression of cardiovascular diseases, moderation is suggested for those who suffer from autoimmune problems or are at a risk of developing them.

Diet is also said to affect the body immunity by directly altering the bacterial population in the gut. Consequently, the regulation of different immune cells occurs. It is well-understood that a Western diet is pro-inflammatory and can have negative effects on the normal microbiota residing in the human gut. Research has shown that bacteria in the gut of people consuming the animal-based Western diet rapidly return to a less inflammatory state by simply adopting a plant-based diet.

Autoimmune Disease and the Modern Food Supply

A less-understood factor that might explain the rapid surge in autoimmune diseases globally is the expansion of choices in the modern food supply. It is suspected that certain food items included in the globalized diet can trigger autoimmune responses. For instance, a study focused on the consumption of cow's milk in children found that it increased their autoimmunity against the cells of the pancreas. This ultimately resulted in an increase of risk for diabetes type 1.

Eventually, it will be possible to connect the DNA of a person to the food that he/she should avoid in order to avoid autoimmune disorders. For now, the best advice is to follow the dietary habits of your ancestors.

Find out where your ancestors — including parents, grandparents, and great-grandparents — from and what types of food did they ate. For example, if a person's ancestors were from Italy, his or her diet would automatically be rich in green beans, tomatoes, olive oil and garbanzo beans. Tomatoes are capable of activating an immune response in a small number of people but there is the remote possibility of them causing autoimmune diseases in the Italians of today. In contrast, a child with Southern Italian or Japanese ancestry would not include milk in their historical diet. Therefore, they are more likely to acquire lactose intolerance in adult life.

If a person has grandparents from Okinawa, he or she is more likely to regularly consume seaweed or sweet potatoes. People with German ancestors are more likely to include asparagus and cabbage in their everyday diet. The process seems complicated but in actuality, it is not. It may require you to have a conversation with your parents or grandparents and ask questions. You can also ask an older person who used to reside in same area as your grandparents. Try to obtain a full list, as every little component of their diet plan was probably to provide total nourishment.

Even if a small village in Italy did not conduct any scientific studies to check which diet was good or bad, everyone knew that the most probable cause of a local B12 deficiency was because they never ate meat, fish or eggs. Similarly, if babies who consumed cow's milk developed certain problems, people would automatically notice it and switch their babies to goat's milk. This type of food selection is easily seen in people residing in small towns and villages but can also occur in cities if the people live in the same place for the majority of their lives. It is more likely to happen in the U.S. or big cities such as Tokyo and London where the communities are transient and people generally do not know about their neighbors' food habits or diseases.

There is no solid evidence that mimicking the dietary habits of your ancestors is going to prevent disease and prolong your life. It is also may not be possible to eat exactly what your parents and grandparents did. Instead, try matching what they ate with the food items included in various dietary interventions such as FMD and the Longevity Diet.

If you do not have the time to wait for the conclusive statements derived from scientific studies and clinical trials, it is completely understandable to adopt the best hypothesis using all the available data. In such a case, the hypothesis is that a town consisting of 2,000 people, together with the surrounding towns, cooperate with the doctors to detect the advantages and disadvantages of particular foods by observing their effects over decades. Most of the data collected this way will definitely be correct. Some portion of it might be incorrect but the risk of taking this approach is zero because the food that your ancestors consumed safely is not going to harm you.

It is also significant to know what your ancestors avoided eating. The market of today might be rich with so-called healthy foods, including kale, quinoa, Curcumin and chia seeds. These foods can definitely provide you with high levels of proteins and vitamins but can be quite harmful to the people whose ancestors never consumed it.

Quinoa, a food originally belonging to the Peruvian Andes, can be safe for the people whose ancestors used it as a staple ingredient. It can also work fine for a vast majority of people across the world. However, quinoa can cause intolerances, allergies and even autoimmune diseases in a small number of people, especially those who are exposed to numerous other risk factors for autoimmune diseases.

For instance, quinoa has shown to increase the immune response in mice. This demonstrates its potential to trigger autoimmune diseases in humans. Quinoa has also been shown to induce allergic reactions in different patients from France and the U.S. So if your ancestors were German, it will better for you to avoid healthy foods such as turmeric and quinoa. These ingredients not a part of the ancient German diet.

FMD and Autoimmune Disease Treatment

FMD has recently been tested for two autoimmune diseases — rheumatoid arthritis and multiple sclerosis. For both diseases, this dietary approach has worked wonders, indicating its potential to reduce the severity of various autoimmune diseases. However, these interventions are still under investigations regarding their efficacy in humans

Multiple Sclerosis

Multiple sclerosis is an autoimmune disease in which the immune cells in your body, particularly the T cells, start attacking the insulating sheath present around the nerve fibers in your central nervous system. The clinical presentation of this disease is frailty of one or more limbs, generalized pain and partial or loss of unilateral vision which may be partial or complete. The patients tend to go through short relapsing episodes of these symptoms. In a few patients, these symptoms can even progress. The role of FMD in preventing and treating multiple sclerosis begun when it was discovered that fasting can significantly decrease the total amount of white blood cells circulating in mice. Moreover, a revival of these cells was observed as soon as the mice resumed eating a normal diet.

In the same study, it was also shown that fasting can activate and even expand the long-term hematopoietic stem cells. This particular form of stem cell can generate different cells of the immune system. Two questions were formulated after this finding:

1. Are dysfunctional cells, including the autoimmune cells, preferentially destroyed by fasting?

2. When humans or animals resume their normal diet after fasting, would the stem cells produce healthy immune cells or autoimmune cells?

The result of the very first set of study including mice was exceptional. It was hypothesized by the scientists that it was essential to kill the autoimmune cells of the body in order to replace them with the normal ones. Therefore, FMD was implemented and it was actually found to work remarkably. FMD cycling not only decreased the severity of multiple sclerosis but also resolved all the symptoms in some of the mice that had already acquired the disease in full form. Every cycle of FMD killed a section of the autoimmune cells whereas three cycles of this disease were able to completely eliminate the problem in about 20 percent of the mice. FMD was also found to work in another amazing way; it enhanced the process of regenerating the damaged myelin in the spinal cord of the mice.

Hence, the FMD cycle was concluded to reverse autoimmunity in mice by destroying the bad autoimmune cells, regenerating the healthy ones and turning on the progenitor cells that can subsequently regenerate the damaged nerves. This has been called as "rejuvenation from within." FMD can kill a lot of cells but it particularly focuses on killing damaged and old immune cells that are no longer able to distinguish between the cells of the body and the invaders such as viruses and bacteria. Fasting can increase stem cells but it reduces the immune cells. After re-feeding, the stem cells produce healthy immune cells.

FMD is said to do a lot more in mice. It prompts their bodies to detect any damage to the spinal cord and immediately turn on the progenitor cells to repair the damage. This leads to one question: Can FMD actually treat multiple sclerosis in humans?

The researchers collaborated to perform a randomized clinical trial on human patients suffering from a relapsing-remitting form of multiple sclerosis. Twenty patients were used for this purpose and were asked to go through a seven-day cycle of FMD, followed by a Mediterranean diet lasting for six months. This was compared with a group of 20 multiple sclerosis patients who continued on a normal diet.

The FMD officially began with a pre-fasting day in which the patients consumed 800 calories coming from rice, fruits and potatoes. This was immediately followed by seven days of fasting during which the patients consumed only 200-to-350 calories per day. The sources of these calories were vegetable juice and vegetable broth supplemented by linseed oil. These juices and broths were consumed three time a day. The patients needed to drink 2-3 liters of unsweetened fluids such as herbal teas and water on a daily basis. After the completion of the seven-day FMD cycle, solid foods were reintroduced slowly. Patients then switched to a plant-based Mediterranean diet for the following six months. Another group of 20 multiple sclerosis patients simultaneously opted for a ketogenic diet for six months as this diet had been previously shown to improve the outcomes in multiple sclerosis.

After the research ended, the patients who received a single cycle of FMD had significantly improved. There was an improvement recorded in their physical health, mental health and the overall quality of life. The side effects not related to multiple sclerosis were found to be similar in all groups and were seen in about 20 percent of the patients placed on a regular diet as well as those undergoing

FMD. The most common side effects were noted to be infections of the respiratory and urinary tract. However, no indication of liver or any other type of damage could be found. Ninety percent of the patients successfully completed their trial. Four relapses in the control group and three in the FMD group were recorded during the six-month study duration.

All in all, the study rendered FMD as a safe and a potentially effective dietary intervention in the patients with multiple sclerosis. However, more extensive studies are still required for the confirmation of results. It is important to note that human subjects received one cycle of FMD as compared to mice that had to go through a number of them. This raises the possibility that the effectiveness of FMD would increase in humans if multiple cycles are tested.

Rheumatoid Arthritis

Rheumatoid arthritis is a chronic inflammatory disease occurring due to the destruction of joints. The disease affects over 1 percent of the overall population and 2 percent of the population over 60 years of age. Consuming a low-calorie diet or fasting lasting for one-to-three weeks has shown to be extremely effective in the treatment of rheumatoid arthritis. The pain and inflammation in rheumatoid arthritis can improve in only five days after the commencement of fasting. However, the symptoms returned as soon as the patients returned to their normal diets. If the fasting period is immediately followed by a vegetable-based diet, some therapeutic effects tend to last. This combination therapy has been used successfully producing results that last for years. The efficiency of this approach has the support of four different studies, two of which were randomized control trials. Fasting has the potential to increase and replace all of the existing medical interventions for a lot of patients who are able to endure it in the long-term.

What is yet to be tried includes multiple or period cycles of FMD conducted every one-to-three months as a treatment of rheumatoid arthritis instead of one cycle followed by dietary changes. Various research-based studies have concluded that the best way to treat rheumatoid arthritis is to opt for FMD cycling, five days per cycle for one-to-three months. Following FMD cycles on a monthly basis has been found to benefit rheumatoid arthritis patients even when there is no switching to a Mediterranean diet in-between. For people who are unable to modify their dietary habits, five days of FMD on a monthly basis will be a good option. The benefit of FMD is that it provides the relatively higher number of calories, which makes it easy for the patients to follow it without the hassle of checking into a clinic.

As per the clinical trials, FMD lasting for seven days has been found to be effective in enhancing the patients' quality of life. Furthermore, a seven-day FMD plan is also more beneficial as compared to a shorter one. Further studies in the future will help the scientists know more about the accurate frequency and length of FMD best suited to treat this disease.

Cancer Cells and the Role of FMD

Immunotherapy is considered as the best and most promising therapy to kill cancer cells and cure cancer. However, studies have shown that FMD can successfully replicate the effects produced by immunotherapy. One particular study explored breast and skin cancer and established that FMD has two important functions that make it a potent therapy for cancer. It can weaken the cancerous cells, remove their protective shield and expose them to immune cells. It can also renew the immune system and increase its aggressiveness towards fighting the cancer.

Chemotherapy-related Steroids and the Role of FMD

Corticosteroids like methylprednisolone, prednisolone and dexamethasone are often used together with chemotherapy to treat cancer. In recent research, it has been shown that dexamethasone increases the glucose levels in blood and causes an increase in the toxicity of a chemotherapy drug, doxorubicin, in mice. By boosting the glucose levels, corticosteroids make the healthy cells of the mice a lot weaker and cancer cells a lot stronger.

This effect was found to be reserved by adding a fasting-mimicking diet as an adjuvant to the chemotherapy. The results indicated that the combination of corticosteroids and chemotherapy must never be used unless there are no suitable alternatives available. In fact, high levels of glucose together with chemotherapy are linked with an increased risk of acquiring infections and an increased death rate as compared to the patients with the blood normal glucose levels. Thus, the current data indicate that steroid hormones can increase the blood glucose level and can be detrimental to health when used in combination with chemotherapy. This called for an alternative treatment for the cancer patients with no other viable options and FMD came as the savior.

The high potential of FMD to treat cancer has rendered it as a "magic shield." It is a dietary modification that can essentially protect people from developing cancer. This claim is supported by science and may clinical trials that are discussed below.

Clinical Trials

One of the earliest clinical trials performed to check the usefulness of FMD in prevention and treatment of cancer involved 18 cancer patients. The participants were placed on a water-only fast that lasted for 24, 48, and 72 hours. This was followed by a platinum-based chemotherapy. As far as the side effects are concerned, 72-hour fasting was found to be linked with more protection as compared to 24-hour fasting. However, the patients found it difficult to follow water-only fasting and therefore, it took almost five years to complete this study.

Another small study involving 13 patients was conducted in Holland. In this study, the participants were placed on a water-only diet for two days and the results were compared to a control group. This study provided results consistent with the previous clinical trial and highlighted the protective benefits of fasting and with respect to the side effects of chemotherapy.

The studies were finally directed towards the benefits of FMD when a university in Berlin tested the effect of a low-calorie FMD diet in 34 women suffering from ovarian and breast cancer. Each woman had received various cycles of chemotherapy with or without fasting. The women who opted for FMD were found to experience a clear-cut reduction in side effects due from chemotherapy.

Numerous clinical trials are still going on and some of them even involve as many as 300 patients. These trials are meant to test the efficiency of a four-day cycle of FMD in combination with regular cancer therapy.

FMD in Cancer Therapy

Extensive testing involving animal models from studies conducted by six laboratories have shown the efficiency of FMD or fasting in protecting the body against the side effects of the standard chemotherapy medicines. These studies have also established how FMD and fasting can increase the effect of regular anti-cancer strategies directed against pancreatic cancer, colorectal cancer, prostate cancer, breast cancer, glioma, neuroblastoma, mesothelioma, lung cancer, melanoma and others. A few small clinical trials and a case series report with 75 patients have provided initial evidence that FMD and fasting are potentially safe and highly effective against the side effects typically seen during chemotherapy sessions. Certain trials are still in process and have tested at least 200 people and provided additional evidence regarding the safety of FMD in chemotherapy as well as its protective effects.

The FMD product meant for cancer patients can be recommended by oncologists after additional tests have been performed and positive results have been obtained. However, the FMD is yet to be proven as a proper method of cancer treatment and must be considered as a part of standard therapies unless it comes to market. It is the right of patients to acquire complete information about the risks of opting a support therapy that is still being tested. Some of the recommendations regarding the FMD to oncologists as well as cancer patients are mentioned below:

1. If the oncologist approves, the patient can adopt the FMD for three days prior to chemotherapy and one day after receiving it. According to the kind of chemotherapy being used and the interval between its cycles, changes can be made in the regimen. Patients must not return to their regular diets unless the chemotherapy falls below the toxic blood levels. This fall is usually observed 24-to-48 hours after the administration.

2. For treatment sessions that last for three days, the patients have an option to adopt the FMD one day before chemotherapy, three days during it, or one-day post-chemotherapy session. The process can be performed for whole five days as well. It is difficult to integrate longer treatment periods with fasting. However, it can be combined with high-calorie FMD after getting an approval from the oncologist.

3. Side effects of FMDs are rarely seen and have only occurred when people have initiated fasting on their own without any medical supervision. In one incidence, a patient caused the liver toxicity markers in his body to increase while fasting on his own and receiving chemotherapy sessions simultaneously. A lot of patients have fainted during hot showers after fasting for multiple days, primarily because of a decrease in their blood glucose levels and blood pressure. Another risk associated with FMD is that immediately returning to normal dietary habits as soon as chemotherapy sessions finish can lead to liver damage. This is because of the combination of certain hepatotoxic drugs and liver cell

proliferation. For this very reason, it is important that the patients wait for at least 24 hours after the last chemotherapy session concludes before returning to a normal diet.

4. Most people can drive safely while they are fasting. Others find no difficulty in operating machinery in this state. However, this is not a universal rule and some people might find it difficult to perform these actions. If you are in doubt, avoid these activities when you are fasting or undergoing an FMD.

5. Starting 24 hours post-chemotherapy, the patient must eat only bread, rice, pasta or a similar source of carbohydrates. They can also consume fruits, vegetables and vegetable soups for 24 hours. Once the required time period (*i.e.* 24 hours) has been completed, the patients can safely resume a normal diet but must pay attention to nourishment like minerals, vitamins, essential fats and proteins.

6. The patients must try their best to maintain their regular body weight before starting another cycle of FMD or fasting

7. As far as the weight loss due to fasting is concerned, obese patients must talk to a qualified doctor and get advice on whether they should maintain their weight or regain what they lost due to fasting.

8. Patients suffering from diabetes must not undergo FMD or fasting unless it has been approved by their endocrinologist or diabetologist.

9. Patients must never fast while they are taking insulin, metformin or drugs with similar effects on the body.

10. Patients who are taking medications for hypertension must talk to their doctor about drops in blood pressure caused by

fasting. They must also discuss all the risks that can occur due to the combination of medications with fasting or FMD.

11. Until the completion of clinical trials, fasting and FMD will remain as experimental procedures and must be considered as a treatment therapy only after getting an approval from oncologists. These procedures must be used along with other standard-of-care therapies. FMD and fasting are to be used as a part of a clinical trial or in conditions where all other interventions have failed to produce any effects.

12. In between the fasting cycles, it is recommended that the cancer patients maintain a low sugar level and consume a plant-based diet with low protein and high nourishment as this diet will allow them to gain and maintain a normal BMI and a healthy weight. A registered dietitian must be consulted in order to prevent malnourishment and unnecessary weight loss.

DIY FMD Meal Plans

In order to follow the FMD to the letter, you have to buy L-Nutra's Prolon products. Disclaimer: Dr. Longo owns equity in L-Nutra via V.D.L. which may raise some eyebrows. However, 100 percent of V.D.L. proceeds are donated to non-profit organizations. This mitigates any potential conflict of interest in the research.

But what if you don't want to buy the Prolon products? Can you still follow the FMD diet?

Obviously, Nutra's ProLon was specifically and scientifically designed to be FMD-compatible. However, if you don't want to buy these products, you can choose to follow one of my meal plans as an alternative. These meal plans have not been tested in a lab environment and they are not exact replicas of the Prolon products.

Alternative meal pans

FMD is a plant-based diet that is designed to attain fasting-like effects while providing micronutrient nourishment such as vitamins, minerals, etc., and minimize the burden of fasting. It comprises of proprietary energy bars, vegetable-based soups, chamomile flower, tea energy drinks, chip snacks and a vegetable supplement formula tablet.

Once a month for five days, participants should limit their calorie intake by 34-54 percent This is low enough to mimic the effects of fasting. For around three weeks of the month, participants should return to their regular eating habits.

FMD consists of a 5-day regime

Phase 1

Moderate protein, high-glycemic, low-fat – days 1 and 2.

Phase 2

High-protein, low-carbohydrate, high-vegetable, low-fat – days 3 and 4.

Phase 3

Moderate-carbohydrate, high healthy fat, moderate protein, hypoglycemic fruit – days 5.

Outlined below are two FMD compatible meal plans.

Meal Plan One

DAY ONE

1,090 calories

★ Breakfast: Black or green tea, 1 slice whole wheat toast (68 calories) and 1 boiled egg (78 calories)

★ Lunch: Tea or black coffee, small green salad with and avocado; dressed with olive oil (300 calories)

★ Snack: 2 almonds (28 calories)

★ Dinner: Mix of green vegetable soup with borlotti beans and 1 slice of whole wheat bread (616 calories)

DAY TWO

725 calories

★ Breakfast: Black or green tea, and 1 poached egg with 1 grilled tomato (100 calories)

★ Lunch: Miso soup (21 calories)

★   Snack: 7 walnut halves (90 calories)

★   Dinner: Vegetable chili with kidney beans and 2 teaspoons of sour cream (514 calories)

DAY THREE

725 calories

★ Breakfast: Black tea, 1 slice whole wheat toast bread with 2 teaspoons of cashew butter (150 calories)

★ Lunch: Espresso, smoked salmon (100g) with watercress (200 calories)

★ Snack: Blueberries (100g) (57 calories)

★ Dinner: Vegetable soup (318 calories)

DAY FOUR

725 calories

★ Breakfast: Black tea, 1 slice of whole wheat toast bread (220 calories) and 1/2 avocado

★ Lunch: Espresso, glass of almond milk (250ml) (60 calories)

★ Snack: 2 squares of 70 percent dark chocolate (110 calories)

★ Dinner: Large green salad with prawns (100g) dressed with olive oil and lemon juice (335 calories)

DAY FIVE

725 calories

★ Breakfast: Black tea and 2 boiled eggs (156 calories).

★ Lunch: Toasted slice with half an avocado and miso soup (210 calories), one apple (60 calories)

★ Dinner: Vegetable soup (large portion) with toasted pine nuts (10g) (299 calories)

Meal Plan Two

DAY ONE

600 calories

★ Breakfast: Mate tea and 1 ripe raw or steamed apple

★ Lunch: Potatoes and vegetables (mostly as soup)

★ Dinner: Potatoes and various vegetables

DAY TWO

700 calories

★ Morning: Warm porridge with fruit as desired and crispbread

★ Lunchtime: Small salad and vegetable risotto

★ Dinner: Vegetable dish with corn or potatoes

DAY THREE

750 calories

★ Breakfast: Muesli with fruit and buttermilk and whole meal bread

★ Lunch: Small salad, vegetables and cereal soup, Quark dessert with fruit

★ Dinner: Small salad, whole meal bread with vegetarian spreads

DAY FOUR

800 calories

★ Breakfast: 1 toasted whole wheat muffin bread with 1 tablespoon of fruit spread, 1 hard-boiled egg and 1 orange

★ Lunch: Bean burrito

★ Dinner: 1 cup zucchini and 1 cup red peppers and 1 small baked potato and 3 ounces baked white fish with lemon juice

DAY FIVE

1,000 calories

★ Breakfast: 2 eggs scrambled (or 1/2 cup egg substitute), 1 slice whole wheat toast bread with 1 teaspoon trans fat-free margarine and 1 small fresh pear (or seasonal fruit)

★ Lunch: 1 cup minestrone, *side salad* with 1 tablespoon low-fat dressing and 1 slice whole grain toast with 1 teaspoon margarine

★ Dinner - 1 1/3 cup beef stew, 1 cup cooked cauliflower and broccoli with

1 tablespoon shredded cheese

Alternative Recipes

Here, I will present a few recipes to give an idea about how to actually do it yourself and not rely on any publications or set menus:

Red Cabbage Salad (ready in 10 minutes)

Ingredients

- 6 ounces red cabbage

- 2 medium-sized carrots

- 1 small avocado

- 1 tablespoon lemon juice

- 1 ounce of apple (shredded)

- ½ cup of cooked corn

- 8 crushed walnuts

Instructions

1. Pulse the cabbage, carrots, and apple in food processor.

2. Cook the corn in the microwave, for 2-3 minutes. Chop the walnuts.

3. Blend the avocado with lemon or lime, adding salt and pepper. Toss all together.

Spicy cauliflower & potatoes (ready in 30 minutes)

Ingredients

- 8 ounces cauliflower

- 6 ounces potatoes

- 1 tablespoon peanut oil

- 6 cashews

- Curry powder and ground turmeric

- Ginger and garlic paste

Instructions

1. In a blender, add the cashews, curry powder and turmeric along with ginger and garlic paste

2. In a pot, heat the peanut oil and add the spice mixture.

3. Next, toss in the cauliflower and potatoes and cover, adding a little more water to prevent the vegetables from sticking. Add salt to taste.

4. Reduce heat and simmer for 20 minutes, lemon juice can be added on top before serving for some fresh taste.

Eggplant Tofu

Ingredients

- 1 small eggplant
- 4 ounces potatoes
- 2 ounces of silken tofu
- 1 tablespoon vegetable oil
- Lemon juice
- Ground turmeric, ground coriander, cayenne pepper
- Salt and pepper
- Fenugreek

Instructions

1. Use the spices to cover the eggplant and potato chunks, use salt and pepper to taste.
2. Use the oil to heat ½ teaspoon fenugreek seeds.
3. Wait until the fenugreek seeds are brown and then add the diced vegetables and cook for 5 minutes.
4. Add ½ cup of water and simmer on low heat for 15-20 minutes.
5. In the last 5 minutes, stir tofu into the mixture.

Off You Go!

You now know how you can achieve the benefits of fasting without having to restrict yourself for long periods. So, there's no more need to deprive yourself of food for long periods of time when you can naturally achieve it by following the Fasting Mimicking Diet. Not only are the health benefits great, but the organization and stability in preparing meals will remove a load of stress. No more wondering about what to eat or which groceries to purchase on your next trip to the store. You can even plan your weekly dishes and prepare them on the weekend. Such organization will save you a lot of time and effort and will make sure that you are sticking with your eating plan at all times.

FMD is a breakthrough that can help you and others to get back in shape and improve your health. FMD protects or simply prevents you from many of the diseases that are can be caused by bad eating habits and a sedentary lifestyle. The best news is, all you need to do is simply comply for a short five days in the beginning and then repeat the cycle after a few months. By making this a habit, you will find yourself on the path of better health and you will enjoy the full life-changing benefits of FMD.

The first few cycles may seem like a stretch, but once you work through the FMD program a few times, it will become much easier. It is a small sacrifice compared to the benefits for your health and waistline. Just follow the tips I shared with you in this book and you'll be A-OK!

Good luck!

One Last Thing... If you enjoyed this book, you can help me tremendously by leaving a review on Amazon. You have no idea how much this would help.

I also want to give you a **one-in-two-hundred chance** to win a **$200.00 Amazon Gift card** as a thank-you for reading this book.

All I ask is that you give me some feedback, so I can improve this or my next book :)

Your opinion is *super valuable* to me. It will only take a minute of your time to let me know what you like and what you didn't like about this book. The hardest part is deciding how to spend the two hundred dollars! Just follow this link.

http://booksfor.review/fmd